* Even if you feel a constant desire to talk about your broken heart with everybody, during this rapid Schock Break Therapy SBT, it is strictly forbidden to talk and even to mention your heart problem! Yes, you think it will discharge the unhappiness in your mind when you talk about your misfortune. But this intuitive thinking is false and it is a trap that all the people fall in! The longer you continue talking about your heart problem the longer you will suffer. That is why, remember, 7 days no talking about your ex! And this Guide helps you not talk and not think about your ex.

***

Afternoon

* Repeat STOP (10 times every 30 min.)

* Say slowly every hour: sun, flower, seven, path, tee, run, yellow, apple, fish, rain, pen, water, smile, talk, life, sky.

* Dinner and half an hour break (you can sleep). Eat at your heart's desire. No diet!

* Nice talk (no complaints) 30 min. When nobody to talk with, phone or internet conversation oral or written with anybody.

* Walk 15 min. With anybody. If nobody to walk with no walk.

* Even if you feel a constant desire to talk about your broken heart with everybody, during this rapid Schock Break Therapy SBT, it is strictly forbidden to talk and even to mention your heart problem! Yes, you think it will discharge the unhappiness in your mind when you talk about your misfortune. But this intuitive thinking is false and it is a trap that all the people fall in! The longer you continue talking about your heart problem the longer you will suffer. That is why, remember, 7 days no talking about your ex! *** and this Guide helps you not talk and not think about your ex.

***

Evening

- Repeat STOP (10 times every 30 min.)
- Say slowly every hour: sun, flower, seven, path, tee, run, yellow, apple, fish, rain, pen, water, smile, talk, life, sky.
- Small supper.
- Nice talk (no complaints) 20 min. When nobody to talk with, phone or internet conversation oral or written with anybody.

The separation with a beloved person is an extremely fragile moment in our life. For many people so much unsupportable that there comes to a very severe psyche crisis when the separation and especially definitive break in a relationship happens. Unfortunately there are hardly any systemic solutions in our societies for this kind of psyche crisis. Even if the suffering is extreme, sometimes even dangerous for the vital survival, people in such a heart trouble do not judge they are psychiatric patients to look for urgent help in a psychiatric hospital. And conversations with a psychologist are not of course sufficient for an urgent and in many cases life threatening moments (the risk of suicide). This Guide will let you survive such difficult moments of your life. Crucial are 7 first days after the separation/break with a beloved person. If you follow this Guide step by step you will survive and come back to a normal and in some time even happy life again!

One thing is very important. Do everything possible to be the first 7 days accompanied by another people, at least one person. It does not have to be anybody close to you. No! It can be a totally strange person. Just anybody you can say „Hello" once a day to. The more poeple in your vicinity the better. When there is no other solution, it is ok to spend the first 7 days in a hotel. There there are always many people. In any case, be NEVER alone the first 7 days after the separation/break.

Day 1

Morning

* If you sleep well and do not have to go to work do not wake up and do not get out of bed early. Sleep as long as you wish, do not rush out of bed.

* Repeat STOP (10 times every 30 min)

* Say slowly every hour: sun, flower, seven, path, tee, run, yellow, apple, fish, rain, pen, water, smile, talk, life, sky.

* Small physical excercise (10 min)

* Breakfast. Eat at your heart's desire. No diet!

* Nice talk (no complaints) 20 min. When nobody to talk with, phone or internet conversation oral or written with anybody.

* Walk 15 min. In anybody's company. If alone, no walk.

- Walk 15 min. With anybody. No walk if nobody to walk with.
- Even if you feel a constant desire to talk about your broken heart with everybody, during this rapid Schock Break Therapy SBT, it is strictly forbidden to talk and even to mention your heart problem! Yes, you think it will discharge the unhappiness in your mind when you talk about your misfortune. But this intuitive thinking is false and it is a trap that all the people fall in! The longer you continue talking about your heart problem the longer you will suffer. That is why, remember, 7 days no talking about your ex! *** and this Guide helps you not talk and not think about your ex.***

Night

Before sleep

- Take a shower (warm water) 1 min.
- Small physical excercise 3 min.

In Bed

- Repeat STOP (20 times)
- Say slowly untill you fall asleep: sun, flower, seven, path, tee, run, yellow, apple, fish, rain, pen, water, smile, talk, life, sky.

If you cannot fall asleep

- Say slowly untill you fall asleep: sun, flower, seven, path, tee, run, yellow, apple, fish, rain, pen, water, smile, talk, life, sky.

If above does not help

- Stand up and go to the toilet (when possible with as little light as possible)
- Say slowly untill you fall asleep: sun, flower, seven, path, tee, run, yellow, apple, fish, rain, pen, water, smile, talk, life, sky.

If above does not help

- Say STOP untill you fall asleep

If above does not help

- Go to the kitchen and have a very small snack.
- Back to the bed say slowly untill you fall asleep: sun, flower, seven, path, tee, run, yellow, apple, fish, rain, pen, water, smile, talk, life, sky.

If above does not help

- Say slowly untill morning: sun, flower, seven, path, tee, run, yellow, apple, fish, rain, pen, water, smile, talk, life, sky.

***

Day 2

Morning

* If you sleep well and do not have to go to work do not wake up and do not get out of bed early. Sleep as long as you wish, do not rush out of bed.

* Repeat STOP (10 times every 30 min)

* Say slowly every hour: sun, flower, seven, path, tee, run, yellow, apple, fish, rain, pen, water, smile, talk, life, sky.

* Small physical excercise (10 min)

* Breakfast. Eat at your heart's desire. No diet!

* Nice talk (no complaints) 20 min. When nobody to talk with, phone or internet conversation oral or written with anybody.

* Walk 15 min. In anybody's company. If alone, no walk.

* Even if you feel a constant desire to talk about your broken heart with everybody, during this rapid Schock Break Therapy SBT, it is strictly forbidden to talk and even to mention your heart problem! Yes, you think it will discharge the unhappiness in your mind when you talk about your misfortune. But this intuitive thinking is false and it is a trap that all the people fall in! The longer you continue talking about your heart problem the longer you will suffer. That is why, remember, 7

days no talking about your ex! And this Guide helps you not talk and not think about your ex.

***

Afternoon

* Repeat STOP (10 times every 30 min.)

* Say slowly every hour: sun, flower, seven, path, tee, run, yellow, apple, fish, rain, pen, water, smile, talk, life, sky.

* Dinner and half an hour break (you can sleep). Eat at your heart's desire. No diet!

* Nice talk (no complaints) 30 min. When nobody to talk with, phone or internet conversation oral or written with anybody.

* Walk 15 min. With anybody. If nobody to walk with no walk.

* Even if you feel a constant desire to talk about your broken heart with everybody, during this rapid Schock Break Therapy SBT, it is strictly forbidden to talk and even to mention your heart problem! Yes, you think it will discharge the unhappiness in your mind when you talk about your misfortune. But this intuitive thinking is false and it is a trap that all the people fall in! The

longer you continue talking about your heart problem the longer you will suffer. That is why, remember, 7 days no talking about your ex! *** and this Guide helps you not talk and not think about your ex.

***

Evening

- Repeat STOP (10 times every 30 min.)
- Say slowly every hour: sun, flower, seven, path, tee, run, yellow, apple, fish, rain, pen, water, smile, talk, life, sky.
- Small supper.
- Nice talk (no complaints) 20 min. When nobody to talk with, phone or internet conversation oral or written with anybody.
- Walk 15 min. With anybody. No walk if nobody to walk with.
- Even if you feel a constant desire to talk about your broken heart with everybody, during this rapid Schock Break Therapy SBT, it is strictly forbidden to talk and even to mention your heart problem! Yes, you think it will discharge the unhappiness in your mind when you

talk about your misfortune. But this intuitive thinking is false and it is a trap that all the people fall in! The longer you continue talking about your heart problem the longer you will suffer. That is why, remember, 7 days no talking about your ex! *** and this Guide helps you not talk and not think about your ex.***

Night

Before sleep

- Take a shower (warm water) 1 min.

- Small physical excercise 3 min.

In Bed

- Repeat STOP (20 times)

- Say slowly untill you fall asleep: sun, flower, seven, path, tee, run, yellow, apple, fish, rain, pen, water, smile, talk, life, sky.

If you cannot fall asleep

- Say slowly untill you fall asleep: sun, flower, seven, path, tee, run, yellow, apple, fish, rain, pen, water, smile, talk, life, sky.

If above does not help

- Stand up and go to the toilet (when possible with as little light as possible)

- Say slowly untill you fall asleep: sun, flower, seven, path, tee, run, yellow, apple, fish, rain, pen, water, smile, talk, life, sky.

If above does not help

- Say STOP untill you fall asleep

If above does not help

- Go to the kitchen and have a very small snack.

- Back to the bed say slowly untill you fall asleep: sun, flower, seven, path, tee, run, yellow, apple, fish, rain, pen, water, smile, talk, life, sky.

If above does not help

- Say slowly untill morning: sun, flower, seven, path, tee, run, yellow, apple, fish, rain, pen, water, smile, talk, life, sky.

***

Day 3

Morning

* If you sleep well and do not have to go to work do not wake up and do not get out of bed early. Sleep as long as you wish, do not rush out of bed.

* Repeat STOP (10 times every 30 min)

* Say slowly every hour: sun, flower, seven, path, tee, run, yellow, apple, fish, rain, pen, water, smile, talk, life, sky.

* Small physical excercise (10 min)

* Breakfast. Eat at your heart's desire. No diet!

* Nice talk (no complaints) 20 min. When nobody to talk with, phone or internet conversation oral or written with anybody.

* Walk 15 min. In anybody's company. If alone, no walk.

* Even if you feel a constant desire to talk about your broken heart with everybody, during this rapid Schock Break Therapy SBT, it is strictly forbidden to talk and even to mention your heart problem! Yes, you think it will discharge the unhappiness in your mind when you talk about your misfortune. But this intuitive thinking is false and it is a trap that all the people fall in! The longer you continue talking about your heart problem the longer you will suffer. That is why, remember, 7 days no talking about your ex! And this Guide helps you not talk and not think about your ex.

***

Afternoon

* Repeat STOP (10 times every 30 min.)

* Say slowly every hour: sun, flower, seven, path, tee, run, yellow, apple, fish, rain, pen, water, smile, talk, life, sky.

* Dinner and half an hour break (you can sleep). Eat at your heart's desire. No diet!

* Nice talk (no complaints) 30 min. When nobody to talk with, phone or internet conversation oral or written with anybody.

* Walk 15 min. With anybody. If nobody to walk with no walk.

* Even if you feel a constant desire to talk about your broken heart with everybody, during this rapid Schock Break Therapy SBT, it is strictly forbidden to talk and even to mention your heart problem! Yes, you think it will discharge the unhappiness in your mind when you talk about your misfortune. But this intuitive thinking is false and it is a trap that all the people fall in! The longer you continue talking about your heart problem the longer you will suffer. That is why, remember, 7 days no talking about your ex! *** and this Guide helps you not talk and not think about your ex.

***

Evening

- Repeat STOP (10 times every 30 min.)

- Say slowly every hour: sun, flower, seven, path, tee, run, yellow, apple, fish, rain, pen, water, smile, talk, life, sky.

- Small supper.

- Nice talk (no complaints) 20 min. When nobody to talk with, phone or internet conversation oral or written with anybody.

- Walk 15 min. With anybody. No walk if nobody to walk with.

- Even if you feel a constant desire to talk about your broken heart with everybody, during this rapid Schock Break Therapy SBT, it is strictly forbidden to talk and even to mention your heart problem! Yes, you think it will discharge the unhappiness in your mind when you talk about your misfortune. But this intuitive thinking is false and it is a trap that all the people fall in! The longer you continue talking about your heart problem the longer you will suffer. That is why, remember, 7 days no talking about your ex! *** and this Guide helps you not talk and not think about your ex.***

Night

Before sleep

- Take a shower (warm water) 1 min.
- Small physical excercise 3 min.

In Bed

- Repeat STOP (20 times)
- Say slowly untill you fall asleep: sun, flower, seven, path, tee, run, yellow, apple, fish, rain, pen, water, smile, talk, life, sky.

If you cannot fall asleep

- Say slowly untill you fall asleep: sun, flower, seven, path, tee, run, yellow, apple, fish, rain, pen, water, smile, talk, life, sky.

If above does not help

- Stand up and go to the toilet (when possible with as little light as possible)
- Say slowly untill you fall asleep: sun, flower, seven, path, tee, run, yellow, apple, fish, rain, pen, water, smile, talk, life, sky.

If above does not help

- Say STOP untill you fall asleep

If above does not help

- Go to the kitchen and have a very small snack.

- Back to the bed say slowly untill you fall asleep: sun, flower, seven, path, tee, run, yellow, apple, fish, rain, pen, water, smile, talk, life, sky.

If above does not help

- Say slowly untill morning: sun, flower, seven, path, tee, run, yellow, apple, fish, rain, pen, water, smile, talk, life, sky.

***

Day 4

Morning

* If you sleep well and do not have to go to work do not wake up and do not get out of bed early. Sleep as long as you wish, do not rush out of bed.

* Repeat STOP (10 times every 30 min)

* Say slowly every hour: sun, flower, seven, path, tee, run, yellow, apple, fish, rain, pen, water, smile, talk, life, sky.

* Small physical excercise (10 min)

* Breakfast. Eat at your heart's desire. No diet!

* Nice talk (no complaints) 20 min. When nobody to talk with, phone or internet conversation oral or written with anybody.

* Walk 15 min. In anybody's company. If alone, no walk.

* Even if you feel a constant desire to talk about your broken heart with everybody, during this rapid Schock Break Therapy SBT, it is strictly forbidden to talk and even to mention your heart problem! Yes, you think it will discharge the unhappiness in your mind when you talk about your misfortune. But this intuitive thinking is false and it is a trap that all the people fall in! The longer you continue talking about your heart problem the longer you will suffer. That is why, remember, 7 days no talking about your ex! And this Guide helps you not talk and not think about your ex.

***

Afternoon

* Repeat STOP (10 times every 30 min.)

* Say slowly every hour: sun, flower, seven, path, tee, run, yellow, apple, fish, rain, pen, water, smile, talk, life, sky.

* Dinner and half an hour break (you can sleep). Eat at your heart's desire. No diet!

* Nice talk (no complaints) 30 min. When nobody to talk with, phone or internet conversation oral or written with anybody.

* Walk 15 min. With anybody. If nobody to walk with no walk.

* Even if you feel a constant desire to talk about your broken heart with everybody, during this rapid Schock Break Therapy SBT, it is strictly forbidden to talk and even to mention your heart problem! Yes, you think it will discharge the unhappiness in your mind when you talk about your misfortune. But this intuitive thinking is false and it is a trap that all the people fall in! The longer you continue talking about your heart problem the longer you will suffer. That is why, remember, 7 days no talking about your ex! *** and this Guide helps you not talk and not think about your ex.

***

Evening

• Repeat STOP (10 times every 30 min.)

• Say slowly every hour: sun, flower, seven, path, tee, run, yellow, apple, fish, rain, pen, water, smile, talk, life, sky.

- Small supper.

- Nice talk (no complaints) 20 min. When nobody to talk with, phone or internet conversation oral or written with anybody.

- Walk 15 min. With anybody. No walk if nobody to walk with.

- Even if you feel a constant desire to talk about your broken heart with everybody, during this rapid Schock Break Therapy SBT, it is strictly forbidden to talk and even to mention your heart problem! Yes, you think it will discharge the unhappiness in your mind when you talk about your misfortune. But this intuitive thinking is false and it is a trap that all the people fall in! The longer you continue talking about your heart problem the longer you will suffer. That is why, remember, 7 days no talking about your ex! *** and this Guide helps you not talk and not think about your ex.***

Night

Before sleep

- Take a shower (warm water) 1 min.

- Small physical excercise 3 min.

In Bed

- Repeat STOP (20 times)

- Say slowly untill you fall asleep: sun, flower, seven, path, tee, run, yellow, apple, fish, rain, pen, water, smile, talk, life, sky.

If you cannot fall asleep

- Say slowly untill you fall asleep: sun, flower, seven, path, tee, run, yellow, apple, fish, rain, pen, water, smile, talk, life, sky.

If above does not help

- Stand up and go to the toilet (when possible with as little light as possible)

- Say slowly untill you fall asleep: sun, flower, seven, path, tee, run, yellow, apple, fish, rain, pen, water, smile, talk, life, sky.

If above does not help

- Say STOP untill you fall asleep

If above does not help

- Go to the kitchen and have a very small snack.

- Back to the bed say slowly untill you fall asleep: sun, flower, seven, path, tee, run, yellow, apple, fish, rain, pen, water, smile, talk, life, sky.

If above does not help

- Say slowly untill morning: sun, flower, seven, path, tee, run, yellow, apple, fish, rain, pen, water, smile, talk, life, sky.

***

Day 5

Morning

* If you sleep well and do not have to go to work do not wake up and do not get out of bed early. Sleep as long as you wish, do not rush out of bed.

* Repeat STOP (10 times every 30 min)

* Say slowly every hour: sun, flower, seven, path, tee, run, yellow, apple, fish, rain, pen, water, smile, talk, life, sky.

* Small physical excercise (10 min)

* Breakfast. Eat at your heart's desire. No diet!

* Nice talk (no complaints) 20 min. When nobody to talk with, phone or internet conversation oral or written with anybody.

* Walk 15 min. In anybody's company. If alone, no walk.

* Even if you feel a constant desire to talk about your broken heart with everybody, during this rapid Schock Break Therapy SBT, it is strictly forbidden to talk and

even to mention your heart problem! Yes, you think it will discharge the unhappiness in your mind when you talk about your misfortune. But this intuitive thinking is false and it is a trap that all the people fall in! The longer you continue talking about your heart problem the longer you will suffer. That is why, remember, 7 days no talking about your ex! And this Guide helps you not talk and not think about your ex.

***

Afternoon

* Repeat STOP (10 times every 30 min.)

* Say slowly every hour: sun, flower, seven, path, tee, run, yellow, apple, fish, rain, pen, water, smile, talk, life, sky.

* Dinner and half an hour break (you can sleep). Eat at your heart's desire. No diet!

* Nice talk (no complaints) 30 min. When nobody to talk with, phone or internet conversation oral or written with anybody.

* Walk 15 min. With anybody. If nobody to walk with no walk.

* Even if you feel a constant desire to talk about your broken heart with everybody, during this rapid Schock Break Therapy SBT, it is strictly forbidden to talk and even to mention your heart problem! Yes, you think it will discharge the unhappiness in your mind when you talk about your misfortune. But this intuitive thinking is false and it is a trap that all the people fall in! The longer you continue talking about your heart problem the longer you will suffer. That is why, remember, 7 days no talking about your ex! *** and this Guide helps you not talk and not think about your ex.

***

Evening

- Repeat STOP (10 times every 30 min.)

- Say slowly every hour: sun, flower, seven, path, tee, run, yellow, apple, fish, rain, pen, water, smile, talk, life, sky.

- Small supper.

- Nice talk (no complaints) 20 min. When nobody to talk with, phone or internet conversation oral or written with anybody.

- Walk 15 min. With anybody. No walk if nobody to walk with.

- Even if you feel a constant desire to talk about your broken heart with everybody, during this rapid Schock Break Therapy SBT, it is strictly forbidden to talk and even to mention your heart problem! Yes, you think it will discharge the unhappiness in your mind when you talk about your misfortune. But this intuitive thinking is false and it is a trap that all the people fall in! The longer you continue talking about your heart problem the longer you will suffer. That is why, remember, 7 days no talking about your ex! *** and this Guide helps you not talk and not think about your ex.***

Night

Before sleep

- Take a shower (warm water) 1 min.

- Small physical excercise 3 min.

In Bed

- Repeat STOP (20 times)

- Say slowly untill you fall asleep: sun, flower, seven, path, tee, run, yellow, apple, fish, rain, pen, water, smile, talk, life, sky.

If you cannot fall asleep

- Say slowly untill you fall asleep: sun, flower, seven, path, tee, run, yellow, apple, fish, rain, pen, water, smile, talk, life, sky.

If above does not help

- Stand up and go to the toilet (when possible with as little light as possible)

- Say slowly untill you fall asleep: sun, flower, seven, path, tee, run, yellow, apple, fish, rain, pen, water, smile, talk, life, sky.

If above does not help

- Say STOP untill you fall asleep

If above does not help

- Go to the kitchen and have a very small snack.

- Back to the bed say slowly untill you fall asleep: sun, flower, seven, path, tee, run, yellow, apple, fish, rain, pen, water, smile, talk, life, sky.

If above does not help

- Say slowly untill morning: sun, flower, seven, path, tee, run, yellow, apple, fish, rain, pen, water, smile, talk, life, sky.

***

Day 6

Morning

* If you sleep well and do not have to go to work do not wake up and do not get out of bed early. Sleep as long as you wish, do not rush out of bed.

* Repeat STOP (10 times every 30 min)

* Say slowly every hour: sun, flower, seven, path, tee, run, yellow, apple, fish, rain, pen, water, smile, talk, life, sky.

* Small physical excercise (10 min)

* Breakfast. Eat at your heart's desire. No diet!

* Nice talk (no complaints) 20 min. When nobody to talk with, phone or internet conversation oral or written with anybody.

* Walk 15 min. In anybody's company. If alone, no walk.

* Even if you feel a constant desire to talk about your broken heart with everybody, during this rapid Schock Break Therapy SBT, it is strictly forbidden to talk and even to mention your heart problem! Yes, you think it will discharge the unhappiness in your mind when you talk about your misfortune. But this intuitive thinking is false and it is a trap that all the people fall in! The longer you continue talking about your heart problem the longer you will suffer. That is why, remember, 7

days no talking about your ex! And this Guide helps you not talk and not think about your ex.

***

Afternoon

* Repeat STOP (10 times every 30 min.)

* Say slowly every hour: sun, flower, seven, path, tee, run, yellow, apple, fish, rain, pen, water, smile, talk, life, sky.

* Dinner and half an hour break (you can sleep). Eat at your heart's desire. No diet!

* Nice talk (no complaints) 30 min. When nobody to talk with, phone or internet conversation oral or written with anybody.

* Walk 15 min. With anybody. If nobody to walk with no walk.

* Even if you feel a constant desire to talk about your broken heart with everybody, during this rapid Schock Break Therapy SBT, it is strictly forbidden to talk and even to mention your heart problem! Yes, you think it will discharge the unhappiness in your mind when you talk about your misfortune. But this intuitive thinking is false and it is a trap that all the people fall in! The

longer you continue talking about your heart problem the longer you will suffer. That is why, remember, 7 days no talking about your ex! *** and this Guide helps you not talk and not think about your ex.

***

Evening

- Repeat STOP (10 times every 30 min.)

- Say slowly every hour: sun, flower, seven, path, tee, run, yellow, apple, fish, rain, pen, water, smile, talk, life, sky.

- Small supper.

- Nice talk (no complaints) 20 min. When nobody to talk with, phone or internet conversation oral or written with anybody.

- Walk 15 min. With anybody. No walk if nobody to walk with.

- Even if you feel a constant desire to talk about your broken heart with everybody, during this rapid Schock Break Therapy SBT, it is strictly forbidden to talk and even to mention your heart problem! Yes, you think it will discharge the unhappiness in your mind when you

talk about your misfortune. But this intuitive thinking is false and it is a trap that all the people fall in! The longer you continue talking about your heart problem the longer you will suffer. That is why, remember, 7 days no talking about your ex! *** and this Guide helps you not talk and not think about your ex.***

Night

Before sleep

- Take a shower (warm water) 1 min.

- Small physical excercise 3 min.

In Bed

- Repeat STOP (20 times)

- Say slowly untill you fall asleep: sun, flower, seven, path, tee, run, yellow, apple, fish, rain, pen, water, smile, talk, life, sky.

If you cannot fall asleep

- Say slowly untill you fall asleep: sun, flower, seven, path, tee, run, yellow, apple, fish, rain, pen, water, smile, talk, life, sky.

If above does not help

- Stand up and go to the toilet (when possible with as little light as possible)

- Say slowly untill you fall asleep: sun, flower, seven, path, tee, run, yellow, apple, fish, rain, pen, water, smile, talk, life, sky.

If above does not help

- Say STOP untill you fall asleep

If above does not help

- Go to the kitchen and have a very small snack.
- Back to the bed say slowly untill you fall asleep: sun, flower, seven, path, tee, run, yellow, apple, fish, rain, pen, water, smile, talk, life, sky.

If above does not help

- Say slowly untill morning: sun, flower, seven, path, tee, run, yellow, apple, fish, rain, pen, water, smile, talk, life, sky.

***

Day 7

Morning

* If you sleep well and do not have to go to work do not wake up and do not get out of bed early. Sleep as long as you wish, do not rush out of bed.

* Repeat STOP (10 times every 30 min)

* Say slowly every hour: sun, flower, seven, path, tee, run, yellow, apple, fish, rain, pen, water, smile, talk, life, sky.

* Small physical excercise (10 min)

* Breakfast. Eat at your heart's desire. No diet!

* Nice talk (no complaints) 20 min. When nobody to talk with, phone or internet conversation oral or written with anybody.

* Walk 15 min. In anybody's company. If alone, no walk.

* Even if you feel a constant desire to talk about your broken heart with everybody, during this rapid Schock Break Therapy SBT, it is strictly forbidden to talk and even to mention your heart problem! Yes, you think it will discharge the unhappiness in your mind when you talk about your misfortune. But this intuitive thinking is false and it is a trap that all the people fall in! The longer you continue talking about your heart problem the longer you will suffer. That is why, remember, 7 days no talking about your ex! And this Guide helps you not talk and not think about your ex.

***

Afternoon

* Repeat STOP (10 times every 30 min.)

* Say slowly every hour: sun, flower, seven, path, tee, run, yellow, apple, fish, rain, pen, water, smile, talk, life, sky.

* Dinner and half an hour break (you can sleep). Eat at your heart's desire. No diet!

* Nice talk (no complaints) 30 min. When nobody to talk with, phone or internet conversation oral or written with anybody.

* Walk 15 min. With anybody. If nobody to walk with no walk.

* Even if you feel a constant desire to talk about your broken heart with everybody, during this rapid Schock Break Therapy SBT, it is strictly forbidden to talk and even to mention your heart problem! Yes, you think it will discharge the unhappiness in your mind when you talk about your misfortune. But this intuitive thinking is false and it is a trap that all the people fall in! The longer you continue talking about your heart problem the longer you will suffer. That is why, remember, 7 days no talking about your ex! *** and this Guide helps you not talk and not think about your ex.

***

Evening

- Repeat STOP (10 times every 30 min.)

- Say slowly every hour: sun, flower, seven, path, tee, run, yellow, apple, fish, rain, pen, water, smile, talk, life, sky.

- Small supper.

- Nice talk (no complaints) 20 min. When nobody to talk with, phone or internet conversation oral or written with anybody.

- Walk 15 min. With anybody. No walk if nobody to walk with.

- Even if you feel a constant desire to talk about your broken heart with everybody, during this rapid Schock Break Therapy SBT, it is strictly forbidden to talk and even to mention your heart problem! Yes, you think it will discharge the unhappiness in your mind when you talk about your misfortune. But this intuitive thinking is false and it is a trap that all the people fall in! The longer you continue talking about your heart problem the longer you will suffer. That is why, remember, 7 days no talking about your ex! *** and this Guide helps you not talk and not think about your ex.***

Night

Before sleep

- Take a shower (warm water) 1 min.
- Small physical excercise 3 min.

In Bed

- Repeat STOP (20 times)
- Say slowly untill you fall asleep: sun, flower, seven, path, tee, run, yellow, apple, fish, rain, pen, water, smile, talk, life, sky.

If you cannot fall asleep

- Say slowly untill you fall asleep: sun, flower, seven, path, tee, run, yellow, apple, fish, rain, pen, water, smile, talk, life, sky.

If above does not help

- Stand up and go to the toilet (when possible with as little light as possible)
- Say slowly untill you fall asleep: sun, flower, seven, path, tee, run, yellow, apple, fish, rain, pen, water, smile, talk, life, sky.

If above does not help

- Say STOP untill you fall asleep

If above does not help

- Go to the kitchen and have a very small snack.

- Back to the bed say slowly untill you fall asleep: sun, flower, seven, path, tee, run, yellow, apple, fish, rain, pen, water, smile, talk, life, sky.

If above does not help

- Say slowly untill morning: sun, flower, seven, path, tee, run, yellow, apple, fish, rain, pen, water, smile, talk, life, sky.

***

Congratulations! You should be proud of yourself! You did it! 7 days! You are saved! Continue next 7 days to make still more progress in recovery.

***

Week Two

***

Day 1

Morning

* If you sleep well and do not have to go to work do not wake up and do not get out of bed early. Sleep as long as you wish, do not rush out of bed.

* Repeat STOP (10 times every 60 min)

* Say slowly every hour: sun, flower, seven, path, tee, run, yellow, apple, fish, rain, pen, water, smile, talk, life, sky.

* Small physical excercise (20 min)

* Breakfast. Eat at your heart's desire. No diet!

* Nice talk (no complaints) 30 min. When nobody to talk with, phone or internet conversation oral or written with anybody.

* Walk 30 min. In anybody's company. If alone, no walk.

* Even if you feel a constant desire to talk about your broken heart with everybody, during this rapid Schock Break Therapy SBT, it is strictly forbidden to talk and even to mention your heart problem! Yes, you think it will discharge the unhappiness in your mind when you talk about your misfortune. But this intuitive thinking is false and it is a trap that all the people fall in! The longer you continue talking about your heart problem the longer you will suffer. That is why, remember, no talking about your ex! And this Guide helps you not talk and not think about your ex.

***

Afternoon

* Repeat STOP (10 times every 60 min.)

* Say slowly every hour: sun, flower, seven, path, tee, run, yellow, apple, fish, rain, pen, water, smile, talk, life, sky.

* Dinner and half an hour break (you can sleep). Eat at your heart's desire. No diet!

* Nice talk (no complaints) 45 min. When nobody to talk with, phone or internet conversation oral or written with anybody.

* Walk 45 min. With anybody. If nobody to walk with no walk.

* Even if you feel a constant desire to talk about your broken heart with everybody, during this rapid Schock Break Therapy SBT, it is strictly forbidden to talk and even to mention your heart problem! Yes, you think it will discharge the unhappiness in your mind when you talk about your misfortune. But this intuitive thinking is false and it is a trap that all the people fall in! The longer you continue talking about your heart problem the longer you will suffer. That is why, remember, no talking about your ex! *** and this Guide helps you not talk and not think about your ex.

***

Evening

- Repeat STOP (10 times every 60 min.)

- Say slowly every hour: sun, flower, seven, path, tee, run, yellow, apple, fish, rain, pen, water, smile, talk, life, sky.

- Small supper.

- Nice talk (no complaints) 45 min. When nobody to talk with, phone or internet conversation oral or written with anybody.

- Walk 30 min. With anybody. No walk if nobody to walk with.

- Even if you feel a constant desire to talk about your broken heart with everybody, during this rapid Schock Break Therapy SBT, it is strictly forbidden to talk and even to mention your heart problem! Yes, you think it will discharge the unhappiness in your mind when you talk about your misfortune. But this intuitive thinking is false and it is a trap that all the people fall in! The longer you continue talking about your heart problem the longer you will suffer. That is why, remember, no talking about your ex! *** and this Guide helps you not talk and not think about your ex.***

Night

Before sleep

- Take a shower (warm water) 1 min.
- Small physical excercise 5 min.

In Bed

- Repeat STOP (20 times)
- Say slowly untill you fall asleep: sun, flower, seven, path, tee, run, yellow, apple, fish, rain, pen, water, smile, talk, life, sky.

If you cannot fall asleep

- Say slowly untill you fall asleep: sun, flower, seven, path, tee, run, yellow, apple, fish, rain, pen, water, smile, talk, life, sky.

If above does not help

- Stand up and go to the toilet (when possible with as little light as possible)
- Say slowly untill you fall asleep: sun, flower, seven, path, tee, run, yellow, apple, fish, rain, pen, water, smile, talk, life, sky.

If above does not help

- Say STOP untill you fall asleep

If above does not help

- Go to the kitchen and have a very small snack.

- Back to the bed say slowly untill you fall asleep: sun, flower, seven, path, tee, run, yellow, apple, fish, rain, pen, water, smile, talk, life, sky.

If above does not help

- Say slowly untill morning: sun, flower, seven, path, tee, run, yellow, apple, fish, rain, pen, water, smile, talk, life, sky.

***

Day 2

Morning

* If you sleep well and do not have to go to work do not wake up and do not get out of bed early. Sleep as long as you wish, do not rush out of bed.

* Repeat STOP (10 times every 60 min)

* Say slowly every hour: sun, flower, seven, path, tee, run, yellow, apple, fish, rain, pen, water, smile, talk, life, sky.

* Small physical excercise (20 min)

* Breakfast. Eat at your heart's desire. No diet!

* Nice talk (no complaints) 30 min. When nobody to talk with, phone or internet conversation oral or written with anybody.

* Walk 30 min. In anybody's company. If alone, no walk.

* Even if you feel a constant desire to talk about your broken heart with everybody, during this rapid Schock Break Therapy SBT, it is strictly forbidden to talk and even to mention your heart problem! Yes, you think it will discharge the unhappiness in your mind when you talk about your misfortune. But this intuitive thinking is false and it is a trap that all the people fall in! The longer you continue talking about your heart problem the longer you will suffer. That is why, remember, no talking about your ex! And this Guide helps you not talk and not think about your ex.

***

Afternoon

* Repeat STOP (10 times every 60 min.)

* Say slowly every hour: sun, flower, seven, path, tee, run, yellow, apple, fish, rain, pen, water, smile, talk, life, sky.

* Dinner and half an hour break (you can sleep). Eat at your heart's desire. No diet!

* Nice talk (no complaints) 45 min. When nobody to talk with, phone or internet conversation oral or written with anybody.

* Walk 45 min. With anybody. If nobody to walk with no walk.

* Even if you feel a constant desire to talk about your broken heart with everybody, during this rapid Schock Break Therapy SBT, it is strictly forbidden to talk and even to mention your heart problem! Yes, you think it will discharge the unhappiness in your mind when you talk about your misfortune. But this intuitive thinking is false and it is a trap that all the people fall in! The longer you continue talking about your heart problem the longer you will suffer. That is why, remember, no talking about your ex! *** and this Guide helps you not talk and not think about your ex.

***

Evening

• Repeat STOP (10 times every 60 min.)

• Say slowly every hour: sun, flower, seven, path, tee, run, yellow, apple, fish, rain, pen, water, smile, talk, life, sky.

- Small supper.

- Nice talk (no complaints) 45 min. When nobody to talk with, phone or internet conversation oral or written with anybody.

- Walk 30 min. With anybody. No walk if nobody to walk with.

- Even if you feel a constant desire to talk about your broken heart with everybody, during this rapid Schock Break Therapy SBT, it is strictly forbidden to talk and even to mention your heart problem! Yes, you think it will discharge the unhappiness in your mind when you talk about your misfortune. But this intuitive thinking is false and it is a trap that all the people fall in! The longer you continue talking about your heart problem the longer you will suffer. That is why, remember, no talking about your ex! *** and this Guide helps you not talk and not think about your ex.***

Night

Before sleep

- Take a shower (warm water) 1 min.

- Small physical excercise 5 min.

In Bed

- Repeat STOP (20 times)

- Say slowly untill you fall asleep: sun, flower, seven, path, tee, run, yellow, apple, fish, rain, pen, water, smile, talk, life, sky.

If you cannot fall asleep

- Say slowly untill you fall asleep: sun, flower, seven, path, tee, run, yellow, apple, fish, rain, pen, water, smile, talk, life, sky.

If above does not help

- Stand up and go to the toilet (when possible with as little light as possible)

- Say slowly untill you fall asleep: sun, flower, seven, path, tee, run, yellow, apple, fish, rain, pen, water, smile, talk, life, sky.

If above does not help

- Say STOP untill you fall asleep

If above does not help

- Go to the kitchen and have a very small snack.

- Back to the bed say slowly untill you fall asleep: sun, flower, seven, path, tee, run, yellow, apple, fish, rain, pen, water, smile, talk, life, sky.

If above does not help

- Say slowly untill morning: sun, flower, seven, path, tee, run, yellow, apple, fish, rain, pen, water, smile, talk, life, sky.

***

Day 3

Morning

* If you sleep well and do not have to go to work do not wake up and do not get out of bed early. Sleep as long as you wish, do not rush out of bed.

* Repeat STOP (10 times every 60 min)

* Say slowly every hour: sun, flower, seven, path, tee, run, yellow, apple, fish, rain, pen, water, smile, talk, life, sky.

* Small physical excercise (20 min)

* Breakfast. Eat at your heart's desire. No diet!

* Nice talk (no complaints) 30 min. When nobody to talk with, phone or internet conversation oral or written with anybody.

* Walk 30 min. In anybody's company. If alone, no walk.

* Even if you feel a constant desire to talk about your broken heart with everybody, during this rapid Schock Break Therapy SBT, it is strictly forbidden to talk and

even to mention your heart problem! Yes, you think it will discharge the unhappiness in your mind when you talk about your misfortune. But this intuitive thinking is false and it is a trap that all the people fall in! The longer you continue talking about your heart problem the longer you will suffer. That is why, remember, no talking about your ex! And this Guide helps you not talk and not think about your ex.

***

Afternoon

* Repeat STOP (10 times every 60 min.)

* Say slowly every hour: sun, flower, seven, path, tee, run, yellow, apple, fish, rain, pen, water, smile, talk, life, sky.

* Dinner and half an hour break (you can sleep). Eat at your heart's desire. No diet!

* Nice talk (no complaints) 45 min. When nobody to talk with, phone or internet conversation oral or written with anybody.

* Walk 45 min. With anybody. If nobody to walk with no walk.

* Even if you feel a constant desire to talk about your broken heart with everybody, during this rapid Schock Break Therapy SBT, it is strictly forbidden to talk and even to mention your heart problem! Yes, you think it will discharge the unhappiness in your mind when you talk about your misfortune. But this intuitive thinking is false and it is a trap that all the people fall in! The longer you continue talking about your heart problem the longer you will suffer. That is why, remember, no talking about your ex! *** and this Guide helps you not talk and not think about your ex.

***

Evening

- Repeat STOP (10 times every 60 min.)
- Say slowly every hour: sun, flower, seven, path, tee, run, yellow, apple, fish, rain, pen, water, smile, talk, life, sky.
- Small supper.
- Nice talk (no complaints) 45 min. When nobody to talk with, phone or internet conversation oral or written with anybody.

- Walk 30 min. With anybody. No walk if nobody to walk with.

- Even if you feel a constant desire to talk about your broken heart with everybody, during this rapid Schock Break Therapy SBT, it is strictly forbidden to talk and even to mention your heart problem! Yes, you think it will discharge the unhappiness in your mind when you talk about your misfortune. But this intuitive thinking is false and it is a trap that all the people fall in! The longer you continue talking about your heart problem the longer you will suffer. That is why, remember, no talking about your ex! and this Guide helps you not talk and not think about your ex.***

Night

Before sleep

- Take a shower (warm water) 1 min.

- Small physical excercise 5 min.

In Bed

- Repeat STOP (20 times)

- Say slowly untill you fall asleep: sun, flower, seven, path, tee, run, yellow, apple, fish, rain, pen, water, smile, talk, life, sky.

If you cannot fall asleep

- Say slowly untill you fall asleep: sun, flower, seven, path, tee, run, yellow, apple, fish, rain, pen, water, smile, talk, life, sky.

If above does not help

- Stand up and go to the toilet (when possible with as little light as possible)

- Say slowly untill you fall asleep: sun, flower, seven, path, tee, run, yellow, apple, fish, rain, pen, water, smile, talk, life, sky.

If above does not help

- Say STOP untill you fall asleep

If above does not help

- Go to the kitchen and have a very small snack.

- Back to the bed say slowly untill you fall asleep: sun, flower, seven, path, tee, run, yellow, apple, fish, rain, pen, water, smile, talk, life, sky.

If above does not help

- Say slowly untill morning: sun, flower, seven, path, tee, run, yellow, apple, fish, rain, pen, water, smile, talk, life, sky.

***

Day 4

Morning

* If you sleep well and do not have to go to work do not wake up and do not get out of bed early. Sleep as long as you wish, do not rush out of bed.

* Repeat STOP (10 times every 60 min)

* Say slowly every hour: sun, flower, seven, path, tee, run, yellow, apple, fish, rain, pen, water, smile, talk, life, sky.

* Small physical excercise (20 min)

* Breakfast. Eat at your heart's desire. No diet!

* Nice talk (no complaints) 30 min. When nobody to talk with, phone or internet conversation oral or written with anybody.

* Walk 30 min. In anybody's company. If alone, no walk.

* Even if you feel a constant desire to talk about your broken heart with everybody, during this rapid Schock Break Therapy SBT, it is strictly forbidden to talk and even to mention your heart problem! Yes, you think it will discharge the unhappiness in your mind when you talk about your misfortune. But this intuitive thinking is false and it is a trap that all the people fall in! The longer you continue talking about your heart problem the longer you will suffer. That is why, remember, no

talking about your ex! And this Guide helps you not talk and not think about your ex.

***

Afternoon

* Repeat STOP (10 times every 60 min.)

* Say slowly every hour: sun, flower, seven, path, tee, run, yellow, apple, fish, rain, pen, water, smile, talk, life, sky.

* Dinner and half an hour break (you can sleep). Eat at your heart's desire. No diet!

* Nice talk (no complaints) 45 min. When nobody to talk with, phone or internet conversation oral or written with anybody.

* Walk 45 min. With anybody. If nobody to walk with no walk.

* Even if you feel a constant desire to talk about your broken heart with everybody, during this rapid Schock Break Therapy SBT, it is strictly forbidden to talk and even to mention your heart problem! Yes, you think it will discharge the unhappiness in your mind when you talk about your misfortune. But this intuitive thinking is false and it is a trap that all the people fall in! The

longer you continue talking about your heart problem the longer you will suffer. That is why, remember, no talking about your ex! and this Guide helps you not talk and not think about your ex.

***

Evening

- Repeat STOP (10 times every 60 min.)
- Say slowly every hour: sun, flower, seven, path, tee, run, yellow, apple, fish, rain, pen, water, smile, talk, life, sky.
- Small supper.
- Nice talk (no complaints) 45 min. When nobody to talk with, phone or internet conversation oral or written with anybody.
- Walk 30 min. With anybody. No walk if nobody to walk with.
- Even if you feel a constant desire to talk about your broken heart with everybody, during this rapid Schock Break Therapy SBT, it is strictly forbidden to talk and even to mention your heart problem! Yes, you think it will discharge the unhappiness in your mind when you

talk about your misfortune. But this intuitive thinking is false and it is a trap that all the people fall in! The longer you continue talking about your heart problem the longer you will suffer. That is why, remember, no talking about your ex! and this Guide helps you not talk and not think about your ex.***

Night

Before sleep

- Take a shower (warm water) 1 min.
- Small physical excercise 5 min.

In Bed

- Repeat STOP (20 times)
- Say slowly untill you fall asleep: sun, flower, seven, path, tee, run, yellow, apple, fish, rain, pen, water, smile, talk, life, sky.

If you cannot fall asleep

- Say slowly untill you fall asleep: sun, flower, seven, path, tee, run, yellow, apple, fish, rain, pen, water, smile, talk, life, sky.

If above does not help

- Stand up and go to the toilet (when possible with as little light as possible)

- Say slowly untill you fall asleep: sun, flower, seven, path, tee, run, yellow, apple, fish, rain, pen, water, smile, talk, life, sky.

If above does not help

- Say STOP untill you fall asleep

If above does not help

- Go to the kitchen and have a very small snack.

- Back to the bed say slowly untill you fall asleep: sun, flower, seven, path, tee, run, yellow, apple, fish, rain, pen, water, smile, talk, life, sky.

If above does not help

- Say slowly untill morning: sun, flower, seven, path, tee, run, yellow, apple, fish, rain, pen, water, smile, talk, life, sky.

***

Day 5

Morning

* If you sleep well and do not have to go to work do not wake up and do not get out of bed early. Sleep as long as you wish, do not rush out of bed.

* Repeat STOP (10 times every 60 min)

* Say slowly every hour: sun, flower, seven, path, tee, run, yellow, apple, fish, rain, pen, water, smile, talk, life, sky.

* Small physical excercise (20 min)

* Breakfast. Eat at your heart's desire. No diet!

* Nice talk (no complaints) 30 min. When nobody to talk with, phone or internet conversation oral or written with anybody.

* Walk 30 min. In anybody's company. If alone, no walk.

* Even if you feel a constant desire to talk about your broken heart with everybody, during this rapid Schock Break Therapy SBT, it is strictly forbidden to talk and even to mention your heart problem! Yes, you think it will discharge the unhappiness in your mind when you talk about your misfortune. But this intuitive thinking is false and it is a trap that all the people fall in! The longer you continue talking about your heart problem the longer you will suffer. That is why, remember, no talking about your ex! And this Guide helps you not talk and not think about your ex.

***

Afternoon

* Repeat STOP (10 times every 60 min.)

* Say slowly every hour: sun, flower, seven, path, tee, run, yellow, apple, fish, rain, pen, water, smile, talk, life, sky.

* Dinner and half an hour break (you can sleep). Eat at your heart's desire. No diet!

* Nice talk (no complaints) 45 min. When nobody to talk with, phone or internet conversation oral or written with anybody.

* Walk 45 min. With anybody. If nobody to walk with no walk.

* Even if you feel a constant desire to talk about your broken heart with everybody, during this rapid Schock Break Therapy SBT, it is strictly forbidden to talk and even to mention your heart problem! Yes, you think it will discharge the unhappiness in your mind when you talk about your misfortune. But this intuitive thinking is false and it is a trap that all the people fall in! The longer you continue talking about your heart problem the longer you will suffer. That is why, remember, no talking about your ex! and this Guide helps you not talk and not think about your ex.

***

Evening

- Repeat STOP (10 times every 60 min.)

- Say slowly every hour: sun, flower, seven, path, tee, run, yellow, apple, fish, rain, pen, water, smile, talk, life, sky.

- Small supper.

- Nice talk (no complaints) 45 min. When nobody to talk with, phone or internet conversation oral or written with anybody.

- Walk 30 min. With anybody. No walk if nobody to walk with.

- Even if you feel a constant desire to talk about your broken heart with everybody, during this rapid Schock Break Therapy SBT, it is strictly forbidden to talk and even to mention your heart problem! Yes, you think it will discharge the unhappiness in your mind when you talk about your misfortune. But this intuitive thinking is false and it is a trap that all the people fall in! The longer you continue talking about your heart problem the longer you will suffer. That is why, remember, no talking about your ex! and this Guide helps you not talk and not think about your ex.***

Night

Before sleep

- Take a shower (warm water) 1 min.
- Small physical excercise 5 min.

In Bed

- Repeat STOP (20 times)
- Say slowly untill you fall asleep: sun, flower, seven, path, tee, run, yellow, apple, fish, rain, pen, water, smile, talk, life, sky.

If you cannot fall asleep

- Say slowly untill you fall asleep: sun, flower, seven, path, tee, run, yellow, apple, fish, rain, pen, water, smile, talk, life, sky.

If above does not help

- Stand up and go to the toilet (when possible with as little light as possible)
- Say slowly untill you fall asleep: sun, flower, seven, path, tee, run, yellow, apple, fish, rain, pen, water, smile, talk, life, sky.

If above does not help

- Say STOP untill you fall asleep

If above does not help

- Go to the kitchen and have a very small snack.

- Back to the bed say slowly untill you fall asleep: sun, flower, seven, path, tee, run, yellow, apple, fish, rain, pen, water, smile, talk, life, sky.

If above does not help

- Say slowly untill morning: sun, flower, seven, path, tee, run, yellow, apple, fish, rain, pen, water, smile, talk, life, sky.

***

Day 6

Morning

* If you sleep well and do not have to go to work do not wake up and do not get out of bed early. Sleep as long as you wish, do not rush out of bed.

* Repeat STOP (10 times every 60 min)

* Say slowly every hour: sun, flower, seven, path, tee, run, yellow, apple, fish, rain, pen, water, smile, talk, life, sky.

* Small physical excercise (20 min)

* Breakfast. Eat at your heart's desire. No diet!

* Nice talk (no complaints) 30 min. When nobody to talk with, phone or internet conversation oral or written with anybody.

* Walk 30 min. In anybody's company. If alone, no walk.

* Even if you feel a constant desire to talk about your broken heart with everybody, during this rapid Schock Break Therapy SBT, it is strictly forbidden to talk and even to mention your heart problem! Yes, you think it will discharge the unhappiness in your mind when you talk about your misfortune. But this intuitive thinking is false and it is a trap that all the people fall in! The longer you continue talking about your heart problem the longer you will suffer. That is why, remember, no talking about your ex! And this Guide helps you not talk and not think about your ex.

***

Afternoon

* Repeat STOP (10 times every 60 min.)

* Say slowly every hour: sun, flower, seven, path, tee, run, yellow, apple, fish, rain, pen, water, smile, talk, life, sky.

* Dinner and half an hour break (you can sleep). Eat at your heart's desire. No diet!

* Nice talk (no complaints) 45 min. When nobody to talk with, phone or internet conversation oral or written with anybody.

* Walk 45 min. With anybody. If nobody to walk with no walk.

* Even if you feel a constant desire to talk about your broken heart with everybody, during this rapid Schock Break Therapy SBT, it is strictly forbidden to talk and even to mention your heart problem! Yes, you think it will discharge the unhappiness in your mind when you talk about your misfortune. But this intuitive thinking is false and it is a trap that all the people fall in! The longer you continue talking about your heart problem the longer you will suffer. That is why, remember, no talking about your ex! and this Guide helps you not talk and not think about your ex.

***

Evening

• 	Repeat STOP (10 times every 60 min.)
• 	Say slowly every hour: sun, flower, seven, path, tee, run, yellow, apple, fish, rain, pen, water, smile, talk, life, sky.

- Small supper.

- Nice talk (no complaints) 45 min. When nobody to talk with, phone or internet conversation oral or written with anybody.

- Walk 30 min. With anybody. No walk if nobody to walk with.

- Even if you feel a constant desire to talk about your broken heart with everybody, during this rapid Schock Break Therapy SBT, it is strictly forbidden to talk and even to mention your heart problem! Yes, you think it will discharge the unhappiness in your mind when you talk about your misfortune. But this intuitive thinking is false and it is a trap that all the people fall in! The longer you continue talking about your heart problem the longer you will suffer. That is why, remember, no talking about your ex! and this Guide helps you not talk and not think about your ex.***

Night

Before sleep

- Take a shower (warm water) 1 min.

- Small physical excercise 5 min.

In Bed

- Repeat STOP (20 times)

- Say slowly untill you fall asleep: sun, flower, seven, path, tee, run, yellow, apple, fish, rain, pen, water, smile, talk, life, sky.

If you cannot fall asleep

- Say slowly untill you fall asleep: sun, flower, seven, path, tee, run, yellow, apple, fish, rain, pen, water, smile, talk, life, sky.

If above does not help

- Stand up and go to the toilet (when possible with as little light as possible)

- Say slowly untill you fall asleep: sun, flower, seven, path, tee, run, yellow, apple, fish, rain, pen, water, smile, talk, life, sky.

If above does not help

- Say STOP untill you fall asleep

If above does not help

- Go to the kitchen and have a very small snack.

- Back to the bed say slowly untill you fall asleep: sun, flower, seven, path, tee, run, yellow, apple, fish, rain, pen, water, smile, talk, life, sky.

If above does not help

- Say slowly untill morning: sun, flower, seven, path, tee, run, yellow, apple, fish, rain, pen, water, smile, talk, life, sky.

***

Day 7

Morning

* If you sleep well and do not have to go to work do not wake up and do not get out of bed early. Sleep as long as you wish, do not rush out of bed.

* Repeat STOP (10 times every 60 min)

* Say slowly every hour: sun, flower, seven, path, tee, run, yellow, apple, fish, rain, pen, water, smile, talk, life, sky.

* Small physical excercise (20 min)

* Breakfast. Eat at your heart's desire. No diet!

* Nice talk (no complaints) 30 min. When nobody to talk with, phone or internet conversation oral or written with anybody.

* Walk 30 min. In anybody's company. If alone, no walk.

* Even if you feel a constant desire to talk about your broken heart with everybody, during this rapid Schock Break Therapy SBT, it is strictly forbidden to talk and

even to mention your heart problem! Yes, you think it will discharge the unhappiness in your mind when you talk about your misfortune. But this intuitive thinking is false and it is a trap that all the people fall in! The longer you continue talking about your heart problem the longer you will suffer. That is why, remember, no talking about your ex! And this Guide helps you not talk and not think about your ex.

***

Afternoon

* Repeat STOP (10 times every 60 min.)

* Say slowly every hour: sun, flower, seven, path, tee, run, yellow, apple, fish, rain, pen, water, smile, talk, life, sky.

* Dinner and half an hour break (you can sleep). Eat at your heart's desire. No diet!

* Nice talk (no complaints) 45 min. When nobody to talk with, phone or internet conversation oral or written with anybody.

* Walk 45 min. With anybody. If nobody to walk with no walk.

* Even if you feel a constant desire to talk about your broken heart with everybody, during this rapid Schock Break Therapy SBT, it is strictly forbidden to talk and even to mention your heart problem! Yes, you think it will discharge the unhappiness in your mind when you talk about your misfortune. But this intuitive thinking is false and it is a trap that all the people fall in! The longer you continue talking about your heart problem the longer you will suffer. That is why, remember, no talking about your ex! and this Guide helps you not talk and not think about your ex.

***

Evening

- Repeat STOP (10 times every 60 min.)
- Say slowly every hour: sun, flower, seven, path, tee, run, yellow, apple, fish, rain, pen, water, smile, talk, life, sky.
- Small supper.
- Nice talk (no complaints) 45 min. When nobody to talk with, phone or internet conversation oral or written with anybody.

- Walk 30 min. With anybody. No walk if nobody to walk with.

- Even if you feel a constant desire to talk about your broken heart with everybody, during this rapid Schock Break Therapy SBT, it is strictly forbidden to talk and even to mention your heart problem! Yes, you think it will discharge the unhappiness in your mind when you talk about your misfortune. But this intuitive thinking is false and it is a trap that all the people fall in! The longer you continue talking about your heart problem the longer you will suffer. That is why, remember, 7 days no talking about your ex! *** and this Guide helps you not talk and not think about your ex.***

Night

Before sleep

- Take a shower (warm water) 1 min.

- Small physical excercise 5 min.

In Bed

- Repeat STOP (20 times)

- Say slowly untill you fall asleep: sun, flower, seven, path, tee, run, yellow, apple, fish, rain, pen, water, smile, talk, life, sky.

If you cannot fall asleep

- Say slowly untill you fall asleep: sun, flower, seven, path, tee, run, yellow, apple, fish, rain, pen, water, smile, talk, life, sky.

If above does not help

- Stand up and go to the toilet (when possible with as little light as possible)
- Say slowly untill you fall asleep: sun, flower, seven, path, tee, run, yellow, apple, fish, rain, pen, water, smile, talk, life, sky.

If above does not help

- Say STOP untill you fall asleep

If above does not help

- Go to the kitchen and have a very small snack.
- Back to the bed say slowly untill you fall asleep: sun, flower, seven, path, tee, run, yellow, apple, fish, rain, pen, water, smile, talk, life, sky.

If above does not help

- Say slowly untill morning: sun, flower, seven, path, tee, run, yellow, apple, fish, rain, pen, water, smile, talk, life, sky.

***

Congratulations! You did it! 14 days! You maybe can already see more colors in life again! If not make one more week of this Rapid Shock Break Therapy.

***

Week Three

***

Day 1

Morning

* If you sleep well and do not have to go to work do not wake up and do not get out of bed early. Sleep as long as you wish, do not rush out of bed.

* Repeat STOP whenever bad thoughts come again.

* Say slowly whenever bad thoughts come again: sun, flower, seven, path, tee, run, yellow, apple, fish, rain, pen, water, smile, talk, life, sky.

* Physical excercise (30 min)

* Breakfast. Eat at your heart's desire. No diet!

* Nice talk (no complaints) 45 min. When nobody to talk with, phone or internet conversation oral or written with anybody.

* Walk 45 min. In anybody's company. If alone, no walk.

* Even if you feel a constant desire to talk about your broken heart with everybody, during this rapid Schock Break Therapy SBT, it is strictly forbidden to talk and even to mention your heart problem! Yes, you think it will discharge the unhappiness in your mind when you talk about your misfortune. But this intuitive thinking is false and it is a trap that all the people fall in! The longer you continue talking about your heart problem the longer you will suffer. That is why, remember, no talking about your ex! And this Guide helps you not talk and not think about your ex.

***

Afternoon

* Repeat STOP (10 times every 60 min.)

* Say slowly every hour: sun, flower, seven, path, tee, run, yellow, apple, fish, rain, pen, water, smile, talk, life, sky.

* Dinner and half an hour break (you can sleep). Eat at your heart's desire. No diet!

* Nice talk (no complaints) 45 min. When nobody to talk with, phone or internet conversation oral or written with anybody.

* Walk 45 min. With anybody. If nobody to walk with no walk.

* Even if you feel a constant desire to talk about your broken heart with everybody, during this rapid Schock Break Therapy SBT, it is strictly forbidden to talk and even to mention your heart problem! Yes, you think it will discharge the unhappiness in your mind when you talk about your misfortune. But this intuitive thinking is false and it is a trap that all the people fall in! The longer you continue talking about your heart problem the longer you will suffer. That is why, remember, no talking about your ex! and this Guide helps you not talk and not think about your ex.

***

Evening

- Repeat STOP whenever bad thoughts come again.
- Say slowly whenever bad thoughts come again: sun, flower, seven, path, tee, run, yellow, apple, fish, rain, pen, water, smile, talk, life, sky.
- Small supper.

- Nice talk (no complaints) 45 min. When nobody to talk with, phone or internet conversation oral or written with anybody.

- Walk 45 min. With anybody. No walk if nobody to walk with.

- Even if you feel a constant desire to talk about your broken heart with everybody, during this rapid Schock Break Therapy SBT, it is strictly forbidden to talk and even to mention your heart problem! Yes, you think it will discharge the unhappiness in your mind when you talk about your misfortune. But this intuitive thinking is false and it is a trap that all the people fall in! The longer you continue talking about your heart problem the longer you will suffer. That is why, remember, no talking about your ex! and this Guide helps you not talk and not think about your ex.***

Night

Before sleep

- Take a shower (warm water) 1 min.

- Small physical excercise 5 min.

In Bed

- Repeat STOP (20 times)

- Say slowly untill you fall asleep: sun, flower, seven, path, tee, run, yellow, apple, fish, rain, pen, water, smile, talk, life, sky.

If you cannot fall asleep

- Say slowly untill you fall asleep: sun, flower, seven, path, tee, run, yellow, apple, fish, rain, pen, water, smile, talk, life, sky.

If above does not help

- Stand up and go to the toilet (when possible with as little light as possible)

- Say slowly untill you fall asleep: sun, flower, seven, path, tee, run, yellow, apple, fish, rain, pen, water, smile, talk, life, sky.

If above does not help

- Say STOP untill you fall asleep

If above does not help

- Go to the kitchen and have a very small snack.

- Back to the bed say slowly untill you fall asleep: sun, flower, seven, path, tee, run, yellow, apple, fish, rain, pen, water, smile, talk, life, sky.

If above does not help

• Say slowly untill morning: sun, flower, seven, path, tee, run, yellow, apple, fish, rain, pen, water, smile, talk, life, sky.

***

Day 2

Morning

* If you sleep well and do not have to go to work do not wake up and do not get out of bed early. Sleep as long as you wish, do not rush out of bed.

* Repeat STOP whenever bad thoughts come again.

* Say slowly whenever bad thoughts come again: sun, flower, seven, path, tee, run, yellow, apple, fish, rain, pen, water, smile, talk, life, sky.

* Physical excercise (30 min)

* Breakfast. Eat at your heart's desire. No diet!

* Nice talk (no complaints) 45 min. When nobody to talk with, phone or internet conversation oral or written with anybody.

* Walk 45 min. In anybody's company. If alone, no walk.

* Even if you feel a constant desire to talk about your broken heart with everybody, during this rapid Schock Break Therapy SBT, it is strictly forbidden to talk and

even to mention your heart problem! Yes, you think it will discharge the unhappiness in your mind when you talk about your misfortune. But this intuitive thinking is false and it is a trap that all the people fall in! The longer you continue talking about your heart problem the longer you will suffer. That is why, remember, no talking about your ex! And this Guide helps you not talk and not think about your ex.

***

Afternoon

* Repeat STOP (10 times every 60 min.)

* Say slowly every hour: sun, flower, seven, path, tee, run, yellow, apple, fish, rain, pen, water, smile, talk, life, sky.

* Dinner and half an hour break (you can sleep). Eat at your heart's desire. No diet!

* Nice talk (no complaints) 45 min. When nobody to talk with, phone or internet conversation oral or written with anybody.

* Walk 45 min. With anybody. If nobody to walk with no walk.

* Even if you feel a constant desire to talk about your broken heart with everybody, during this rapid Schock Break Therapy SBT, it is strictly forbidden to talk and even to mention your heart problem! Yes, you think it will discharge the unhappiness in your mind when you talk about your misfortune. But this intuitive thinking is false and it is a trap that all the people fall in! The longer you continue talking about your heart problem the longer you will suffer. That is why, remember, no talking about your ex! and this Guide helps you not talk and not think about your ex.

***

Evening

- Repeat STOP whenever bad thoughts come again.
- Say slowly whenever bad thoughts come again: sun, flower, seven, path, tee, run, yellow, apple, fish, rain, pen, water, smile, talk, life, sky.
- Small supper.
- Nice talk (no complaints) 45 min. When nobody to talk with, phone or internet conversation oral or written with anybody.

- Walk 45 min. With anybody. No walk if nobody to walk with.

- Even if you feel a constant desire to talk about your broken heart with everybody, during this rapid Schock Break Therapy SBT, it is strictly forbidden to talk and even to mention your heart problem! Yes, you think it will discharge the unhappiness in your mind when you talk about your misfortune. But this intuitive thinking is false and it is a trap that all the people fall in! The longer you continue talking about your heart problem the longer you will suffer. That is why, remember, no talking about your ex! and this Guide helps you not talk and not think about your ex.***

Night

Before sleep

- Take a shower (warm water) 1 min.

- Small physical excercise 5 min.

In Bed

- Repeat STOP (20 times)

- Say slowly untill you fall asleep: sun, flower, seven, path, tee, run, yellow, apple, fish, rain, pen, water, smile, talk, life, sky.

If you cannot fall asleep

- Say slowly untill you fall asleep: sun, flower, seven, path, tee, run, yellow, apple, fish, rain, pen, water, smile, talk, life, sky.

If above does not help

- Stand up and go to the toilet (when possible with as little light as possible)

- Say slowly untill you fall asleep: sun, flower, seven, path, tee, run, yellow, apple, fish, rain, pen, water, smile, talk, life, sky.

If above does not help

- Say STOP untill you fall asleep

If above does not help

- Go to the kitchen and have a very small snack.

- Back to the bed say slowly untill you fall asleep: sun, flower, seven, path, tee, run, yellow, apple, fish, rain, pen, water, smile, talk, life, sky.

If above does not help

- Say slowly untill morning: sun, flower, seven, path, tee, run, yellow, apple, fish, rain, pen, water, smile, talk, life, sky.

***

Day 3

Morning

* If you sleep well and do not have to go to work do not wake up and do not get out of bed early. Sleep as long as you wish, do not rush out of bed.

* Repeat STOP whenever bad thoughts come again.

* Say slowly whenever bad thoughts come again: sun, flower, seven, path, tee, run, yellow, apple, fish, rain, pen, water, smile, talk, life, sky.

* Physical excercise (30 min)

* Breakfast. Eat at your heart's desire. No diet!

* Nice talk (no complaints) 45 min. When nobody to talk with, phone or internet conversation oral or written with anybody.

* Walk 45 min. In anybody's company. If alone, no walk.

* Even if you feel a constant desire to talk about your broken heart with everybody, during this rapid Schock Break Therapy SBT, it is strictly forbidden to talk and even to mention your heart problem! Yes, you think it will discharge the unhappiness in your mind when you talk about your misfortune. But this intuitive thinking is false and it is a trap that all the people fall in! The longer you continue talking about your heart problem the longer you will suffer. That is why, remember, no

talking about your ex! And this Guide helps you not talk and not think about your ex.

***

Afternoon

* Repeat STOP (10 times every 60 min.)

* Say slowly every hour: sun, flower, seven, path, tee, run, yellow, apple, fish, rain, pen, water, smile, talk, life, sky.

* Dinner and half an hour break (you can sleep). Eat at your heart's desire. No diet!

* Nice talk (no complaints) 45 min. When nobody to talk with, phone or internet conversation oral or written with anybody.

* Walk 45 min. With anybody. If nobody to walk with no walk.

* Even if you feel a constant desire to talk about your broken heart with everybody, during this rapid Schock Break Therapy SBT, it is strictly forbidden to talk and even to mention your heart problem! Yes, you think it will discharge the unhappiness in your mind when you talk about your misfortune. But this intuitive thinking is false and it is a trap that all the people fall in! The

longer you continue talking about your heart problem the longer you will suffer. That is why, remember, no talking about your ex! and this Guide helps you not talk and not think about your ex.

***

Evening

- Repeat STOP whenever bad thoughts come again.
- Say slowly whenever bad thoughts come again: sun, flower, seven, path, tee, run, yellow, apple, fish, rain, pen, water, smile, talk, life, sky.
- Small supper.
- Nice talk (no complaints) 45 min. When nobody to talk with, phone or internet conversation oral or written with anybody.
- Walk 45 min. With anybody. No walk if nobody to walk with.
- Even if you feel a constant desire to talk about your broken heart with everybody, during this rapid Schock Break Therapy SBT, it is strictly forbidden to talk and even to mention your heart problem! Yes, you think it will discharge the unhappiness in your mind when you

talk about your misfortune. But this intuitive thinking is false and it is a trap that all the people fall in! The longer you continue talking about your heart problem the longer you will suffer. That is why, remember, no talking about your ex! and this Guide helps you not talk and not think about your ex.***

Night

Before sleep

- Take a shower (warm water) 1 min.

- Small physical excercise 5 min.

In Bed

- Repeat STOP (20 times)

- Say slowly untill you fall asleep: sun, flower, seven, path, tee, run, yellow, apple, fish, rain, pen, water, smile, talk, life, sky.

If you cannot fall asleep

- Say slowly untill you fall asleep: sun, flower, seven, path, tee, run, yellow, apple, fish, rain, pen, water, smile, talk, life, sky.

If above does not help

- Stand up and go to the toilet (when possible with as little light as possible)

- Say slowly untill you fall asleep: sun, flower, seven, path, tee, run, yellow, apple, fish, rain, pen, water, smile, talk, life, sky.

If above does not help

- Say STOP untill you fall asleep

If above does not help

- Go to the kitchen and have a very small snack.

- Back to the bed say slowly untill you fall asleep: sun, flower, seven, path, tee, run, yellow, apple, fish, rain, pen, water, smile, talk, life, sky.

If above does not help

- Say slowly untill morning: sun, flower, seven, path, tee, run, yellow, apple, fish, rain, pen, water, smile, talk, life, sky.

***

Day 4

Morning

* If you sleep well and do not have to go to work do not wake up and do not get out of bed early. Sleep as long as you wish, do not rush out of bed.

* Repeat STOP whenever bad thoughts come again.

* Say slowly whenever bad thoughts come again: sun, flower, seven, path, tee, run, yellow, apple, fish, rain, pen, water, smile, talk, life, sky.

* Physical excercise (30 min)

* Breakfast. Eat at your heart's desire. No diet!

* Nice talk (no complaints) 45 min. When nobody to talk with, phone or internet conversation oral or written with anybody.

* Walk 45 min. In anybody's company. If alone, no walk.

* Even if you feel a constant desire to talk about your broken heart with everybody, during this rapid Schock Break Therapy SBT, it is strictly forbidden to talk and even to mention your heart problem! Yes, you think it will discharge the unhappiness in your mind when you talk about your misfortune. But this intuitive thinking is false and it is a trap that all the people fall in! The longer you continue talking about your heart problem the longer you will suffer. That is why, remember, no talking about your ex! And this Guide helps you not talk and not think about your ex.

***

Afternoon

* Repeat STOP (10 times every 60 min.)

* Say slowly every hour: sun, flower, seven, path, tee, run, yellow, apple, fish, rain, pen, water, smile, talk, life, sky.

* Dinner and half an hour break (you can sleep). Eat at your heart's desire. No diet!

* Nice talk (no complaints) 45 min. When nobody to talk with, phone or internet conversation oral or written with anybody.

* Walk 45 min. With anybody. If nobody to walk with no walk.

* Even if you feel a constant desire to talk about your broken heart with everybody, during this rapid Schock Break Therapy SBT, it is strictly forbidden to talk and even to mention your heart problem! Yes, you think it will discharge the unhappiness in your mind when you talk about your misfortune. But this intuitive thinking is false and it is a trap that all the people fall in! The longer you continue talking about your heart problem the longer you will suffer. That is why, remember, no talking about your ex! and this Guide helps you not talk and not think about your ex.

***

Evening

- Repeat STOP whenever bad thoughts come again.

- Say slowly whenever bad thoughts come again: sun, flower, seven, path, tee, run, yellow, apple, fish, rain, pen, water, smile, talk, life, sky.

- Small supper.

- Nice talk (no complaints) 45 min. When nobody to talk with, phone or internet conversation oral or written with anybody.

- Walk 45 min. With anybody. No walk if nobody to walk with.

- Even if you feel a constant desire to talk about your broken heart with everybody, during this rapid Schock Break Therapy SBT, it is strictly forbidden to talk and even to mention your heart problem! Yes, you think it will discharge the unhappiness in your mind when you talk about your misfortune. But this intuitive thinking is false and it is a trap that all the people fall in! The longer you continue talking about your heart problem the longer you will suffer. That is why, remember, no talking about your ex! and this Guide helps you not talk and not think about your ex.***

Night

Before sleep

- Take a shower (warm water) 1 min.

- Small physical excercise 5 min.

In Bed

- Repeat STOP (20 times)

- Say slowly untill you fall asleep: sun, flower, seven, path, tee, run, yellow, apple, fish, rain, pen, water, smile, talk, life, sky.

If you cannot fall asleep

- Say slowly untill you fall asleep: sun, flower, seven, path, tee, run, yellow, apple, fish, rain, pen, water, smile, talk, life, sky.

If above does not help

- Stand up and go to the toilet (when possible with as little light as possible)

- Say slowly untill you fall asleep: sun, flower, seven, path, tee, run, yellow, apple, fish, rain, pen, water, smile, talk, life, sky.

If above does not help

- Say STOP untill you fall asleep

If above does not help

- Go to the kitchen and have a very small snack.

- Back to the bed say slowly untill you fall asleep: sun, flower, seven, path, tee, run, yellow, apple, fish, rain, pen, water, smile, talk, life, sky.

If above does not help

- Say slowly untill morning: sun, flower, seven, path, tee, run, yellow, apple, fish, rain, pen, water, smile, talk, life, sky.

***

Day 5

Morning

* If you sleep well and do not have to go to work do not wake up and do not get out of bed early. Sleep as long as you wish, do not rush out of bed.

* Repeat STOP whenever bad thoughts come again.

* Say slowly whenever bad thoughts come again: sun, flower, seven, path, tee, run, yellow, apple, fish, rain, pen, water, smile, talk, life, sky.

* Physical excercise (30 min)

* Breakfast. Eat at your heart's desire. No diet!

* Nice talk (no complaints) 45 min. When nobody to talk with, phone or internet conversation oral or written with anybody.

* Walk 45 min. In anybody's company. If alone, no walk.

* Even if you feel a constant desire to talk about your broken heart with everybody, during this rapid Schock Break Therapy SBT, it is strictly forbidden to talk and even to mention your heart problem! Yes, you think it will discharge the unhappiness in your mind when you talk about your misfortune. But this intuitive thinking is false and it is a trap that all the people fall in! The longer you continue talking about your heart problem the longer you will suffer. That is why, remember, no talking about your ex! And this Guide helps you not talk and not think about your ex.

***

Afternoon

* Repeat STOP (10 times every 60 min.)

* Say slowly every hour: sun, flower, seven, path, tee, run, yellow, apple, fish, rain, pen, water, smile, talk, life, sky.

* Dinner and half an hour break (you can sleep). Eat at your heart's desire. No diet!

* Nice talk (no complaints) 45 min. When nobody to talk with, phone or internet conversation oral or written with anybody.

* Walk 45 min. With anybody. If nobody to walk with no walk.

* Even if you feel a constant desire to talk about your broken heart with everybody, during this rapid Schock Break Therapy SBT, it is strictly forbidden to talk and even to mention your heart problem! Yes, you think it will discharge the unhappiness in your mind when you talk about your misfortune. But this intuitive thinking is false and it is a trap that all the people fall in! The longer you continue talking about your heart problem the longer you will suffer. That is why, remember, no talking about your ex! and this Guide helps you not talk and not think about your ex.

***

Evening

- Repeat STOP whenever bad thoughts come again.
- Say slowly whenever bad thoughts come again: sun, flower, seven, path, tee, run, yellow, apple, fish, rain, pen, water, smile, talk, life, sky.

- Small supper.

- Nice talk (no complaints) 45 min. When nobody to talk with, phone or internet conversation oral or written with anybody.

- Walk 45 min. With anybody. No walk if nobody to walk with.

- Even if you feel a constant desire to talk about your broken heart with everybody, during this rapid Schock Break Therapy SBT, it is strictly forbidden to talk and even to mention your heart problem! Yes, you think it will discharge the unhappiness in your mind when you talk about your misfortune. But this intuitive thinking is false and it is a trap that all the people fall in! The longer you continue talking about your heart problem the longer you will suffer. That is why, remember, no talking about your ex! and this Guide helps you not talk and not think about your ex.***

Night

Before sleep

- Take a shower (warm water) 1 min.

- Small physical excercise 5 min.

In Bed

- Repeat STOP (20 times)

- Say slowly untill you fall asleep: sun, flower, seven, path, tee, run, yellow, apple, fish, rain, pen, water, smile, talk, life, sky.

If you cannot fall asleep

- Say slowly untill you fall asleep: sun, flower, seven, path, tee, run, yellow, apple, fish, rain, pen, water, smile, talk, life, sky.

If above does not help

- Stand up and go to the toilet (when possible with as little light as possible)

- Say slowly untill you fall asleep: sun, flower, seven, path, tee, run, yellow, apple, fish, rain, pen, water, smile, talk, life, sky.

If above does not help

- Say STOP untill you fall asleep

If above does not help

- Go to the kitchen and have a very small snack.

- Back to the bed say slowly untill you fall asleep: sun, flower, seven, path, tee, run, yellow, apple, fish, rain, pen, water, smile, talk, life, sky.

If above does not help

- Say slowly untill morning: sun, flower, seven, path, tee, run, yellow, apple, fish, rain, pen, water, smile, talk, life, sky.

***

Day 6

Morning

* If you sleep well and do not have to go to work do not wake up and do not get out of bed early. Sleep as long as you wish, do not rush out of bed.

* Repeat STOP whenever bad thoughts come again.

* Say slowly whenever bad thoughts come again: sun, flower, seven, path, tee, run, yellow, apple, fish, rain, pen, water, smile, talk, life, sky.

* Physical excercise (30 min)

* Breakfast. Eat at your heart's desire. No diet!

* Nice talk (no complaints) 45 min. When nobody to talk with, phone or internet conversation oral or written with anybody.

* Walk 45 min. In anybody's company. If alone, no walk.

* Even if you feel a constant desire to talk about your broken heart with everybody, during this rapid Schock Break Therapy SBT, it is strictly forbidden to talk and

even to mention your heart problem! Yes, you think it will discharge the unhappiness in your mind when you talk about your misfortune. But this intuitive thinking is false and it is a trap that all the people fall in! The longer you continue talking about your heart problem the longer you will suffer. That is why, remember, no talking about your ex! And this Guide helps you not talk and not think about your ex.

***

Afternoon

* Repeat STOP (10 times every 60 min.)

* Say slowly every hour: sun, flower, seven, path, tee, run, yellow, apple, fish, rain, pen, water, smile, talk, life, sky.

* Dinner and half an hour break (you can sleep). Eat at your heart's desire. No diet!

* Nice talk (no complaints) 45 min. When nobody to talk with, phone or internet conversation oral or written with anybody.

* Walk 45 min. With anybody. If nobody to walk with no walk.

* Even if you feel a constant desire to talk about your broken heart with everybody, during this rapid Schock Break Therapy SBT, it is strictly forbidden to talk and even to mention your heart problem! Yes, you think it will discharge the unhappiness in your mind when you talk about your misfortune. But this intuitive thinking is false and it is a trap that all the people fall in! The longer you continue talking about your heart problem the longer you will suffer. That is why, remember, no talking about your ex! and this Guide helps you not talk and not think about your ex.

***

Evening

• Repeat STOP whenever bad thoughts come again.

• Say slowly whenever bad thoughts come again: sun, flower, seven, path, tee, run, yellow, apple, fish, rain, pen, water, smile, talk, life, sky.

• Small supper.

• Nice talk (no complaints) 45 min. When nobody to talk with, phone or internet conversation oral or written with anybody.

- Walk 45 min. With anybody. No walk if nobody to walk with.

- Even if you feel a constant desire to talk about your broken heart with everybody, during this rapid Schock Break Therapy SBT, it is strictly forbidden to talk and even to mention your heart problem! Yes, you think it will discharge the unhappiness in your mind when you talk about your misfortune. But this intuitive thinking is false and it is a trap that all the people fall in! The longer you continue talking about your heart problem the longer you will suffer. That is why, remember, no talking about your ex! and this Guide helps you not talk and not think about your ex.***

Night

Before sleep

- Take a shower (warm water) 1 min.

- Small physical excercise 5 min.

In Bed

- Repeat STOP (20 times)

- Say slowly untill you fall asleep: sun, flower, seven, path, tee, run, yellow, apple, fish, rain, pen, water, smile, talk, life, sky.

If you cannot fall asleep

- Say slowly untill you fall asleep: sun, flower, seven, path, tee, run, yellow, apple, fish, rain, pen, water, smile, talk, life, sky.

If above does not help

- Stand up and go to the toilet (when possible with as little light as possible)

- Say slowly untill you fall asleep: sun, flower, seven, path, tee, run, yellow, apple, fish, rain, pen, water, smile, talk, life, sky.

If above does not help

- Say STOP untill you fall asleep

If above does not help

- Go to the kitchen and have a very small snack.

- Back to the bed say slowly untill you fall asleep: sun, flower, seven, path, tee, run, yellow, apple, fish, rain, pen, water, smile, talk, life, sky.

If above does not help

- Say slowly untill morning: sun, flower, seven, path, tee, run, yellow, apple, fish, rain, pen, water, smile, talk, life, sky.

***

Day 7

Morning

* If you sleep well and do not have to go to work do not wake up and do not get out of bed early. Sleep as long as you wish, do not rush out of bed.

* Repeat STOP whenever bad thoughts come again.

* Say slowly whenever bad thoughts come again: sun, flower, seven, path, tee, run, yellow, apple, fish, rain, pen, water, smile, talk, life, sky.

* Physical excercise (30 min)

* Breakfast. Eat at your heart's desire. No diet!

* Nice talk (no complaints) 45 min. When nobody to talk with, phone or internet conversation oral or written with anybody.

* Walk 45 min. In anybody's company. If alone, no walk.

* Even if you feel a constant desire to talk about your broken heart with everybody, during this rapid Schock Break Therapy SBT, it is strictly forbidden to talk and even to mention your heart problem! Yes, you think it will discharge the unhappiness in your mind when you talk about your misfortune. But this intuitive thinking is false and it is a trap that all the people fall in! The longer you continue talking about your heart problem the longer you will suffer. That is why, remember, no

talking about your ex! And this Guide helps you not talk and not think about your ex.

***

Afternoon

* Repeat STOP (10 times every 60 min.)

* Say slowly every hour: sun, flower, seven, path, tee, run, yellow, apple, fish, rain, pen, water, smile, talk, life, sky.

* Dinner and half an hour break (you can sleep). Eat at your heart's desire. No diet!

* Nice talk (no complaints) 45 min. When nobody to talk with, phone or internet conversation oral or written with anybody.

* Walk 45 min. With anybody. If nobody to walk with no walk.

* Even if you feel a constant desire to talk about your broken heart with everybody, during this rapid Schock Break Therapy SBT, it is strictly forbidden to talk and even to mention your heart problem! Yes, you think it will discharge the unhappiness in your mind when you talk about your misfortune. But this intuitive thinking is false and it is a trap that all the people fall in! The

longer you continue talking about your heart problem the longer you will suffer. That is why, remember, no talking about your ex! and this Guide helps you not talk and not think about your ex.

***

Evening

- Repeat STOP whenever bad thoughts come again.

- Say slowly whenever bad thoughts come again: sun, flower, seven, path, tee, run, yellow, apple, fish, rain, pen, water, smile, talk, life, sky.

- Small supper.

- Nice talk (no complaints) 45 min. When nobody to talk with, phone or internet conversation oral or written with anybody.

- Walk 45 min. With anybody. No walk if nobody to walk with.

- Even if you feel a constant desire to talk about your broken heart with everybody, during this rapid Schock Break Therapy SBT, it is strictly forbidden to talk and even to mention your heart problem! Yes, you think it will discharge the unhappiness in your mind when you

talk about your misfortune. But this intuitive thinking is false and it is a trap that all the people fall in! The longer you continue talking about your heart problem the longer you will suffer. That is why, remember, no talking about your ex! and this Guide helps you not talk and not think about your ex.***

Night

Before sleep

- Take a shower (warm water) 1 min.

- Small physical excercise 5 min.

In Bed

- Repeat STOP (20 times)

- Say slowly untill you fall asleep: sun, flower, seven, path, tee, run, yellow, apple, fish, rain, pen, water, smile, talk, life, sky.

If you cannot fall asleep

- Say slowly untill you fall asleep: sun, flower, seven, path, tee, run, yellow, apple, fish, rain, pen, water, smile, talk, life, sky.

If above does not help

- Stand up and go to the toilet (when possible with as little light as possible)

- Say slowly untill you fall asleep: sun, flower, seven, path, tee, run, yellow, apple, fish, rain, pen, water, smile, talk, life, sky.

If above does not help

- Say STOP untill you fall asleep

If above does not help

- Go to the kitchen and have a very small snack.

- Back to the bed say slowly untill you fall asleep: sun, flower, seven, path, tee, run, yellow, apple, fish, rain, pen, water, smile, talk, life, sky.

If above does not help

- Say slowly untill morning: sun, flower, seven, path, tee, run, yellow, apple, fish, rain, pen, water, smile, talk, life, sky.

***

Congratulations! 3 weeks RSBT Therapy behind you and you can enjoy your life again. In a case you still feel some psyche discomfort continue the RSBT week after week following the pattern week 3 untill you are totally recovered.

www.ingramcontent.com/pod-product-compliance
Lightning Source LLC
Chambersburg PA
CBHW070111230526
45472CB00004B/1210